The Flexible Struggle

Navigating Life with Ehlers-Danlos Syndrome

By

Gregory H. Cayer

Table of content

This book is dedicated to all people who have shown steadfast resilience in the face of Ehlers-Danlos syndrome, to the resilient individuals who inspire us with their bravery, and to the caring families and friends who give unwavering support.

May this book serve as a guiding light, a source of information, and a monument to the power of community. Together, we navigate the flexible struggle, accepting life's problems with grace, persistence, and the steadfast hope that a greater, more compassionate future awaits.

About the author

Gregory H. Cayer is not only a writer, he's a sympathetic guide through the nuanced journey of "The Flexible Struggle: Navigating Life with Ehlers-Danlos Syndrome." With a genuine devotion to understanding the human experience, Gregory's words in this book offer a lifeline for people experiencing the specific difficulties of EDS.

Through his work, he encourages readers to accompany him on a transformational adventure, exploring the perseverance and fortitude of those contending with Ehlers-Danlos syndrome. Gregory's thoughts and narrative skills clarify the way, bringing consolation, empowerment, and a greater knowledge of the adaptable battle.

Gregory H. Cayer's work is not simply literature; it's a monument to the lasting spirit of individuals living with EDS and a source of inspiration for anybody attempting to face life's problems with grace and bravery. In "The Flexible Struggle," his words become a light of hope, leading readers through the maze of EDS with empathy, knowledge, and unflinching support.

In the tapestry of life, we frequently find ourselves confronting unique obstacles, and for some, the path takes an exceptional turn. "The Flexible Struggle: Navigating Life with Ehlers-Danlos Syndrome" is a testimonial to the tenacious human spirit in the face of a unique and difficult affliction.

Within these pages, we begin a comprehensive investigation of Ehlers-Danlos syndrome (EDS), a disorder that pushes the boundaries of resilience and flexibility. EDS, marked by hypermobility, fragility, and unpredictability, is not only a medical diagnosis; it is a deep life experience.

As we go into this book, we delve into the tales of people who fight EDS every day. Their experiences, their obstacles, and their achievements serve as a tribute to the power of the human spirit. Each page provides insights, practical assistance, and, most importantly, a feeling of connection to people who deal with EDS.

"The Flexible Struggle" is more than a book; it is a light of understanding, empathy, and hope. It is a guide through the convoluted roads of EDS, a source of information for the inquisitive, and a refuge of support for those in need.

Join us on this incredible journey—one that shows not only the struggle but also the tenacity, fortitude, and adaptation that characterize the human experience. In these tales, you will find peace, inspiration, and a poignant reminder that even in the midst of life's most difficult obstacles, the human spirit remains unquestionably adaptable.

Chapter 1

History Of Ehlers Danlos Syndrome

The tale of Ehlers-Danlos Syndrome (EDS) spans more than a century and is one of medical curiosity, persistence, and scientific discovery. The two physicians Edvard Ehlers and Henri-Alexandre Danlos, who significantly contributed to the knowledge of the disease, gave it their names. Here is a more thorough look at the Ehlers-Danlos Syndrome's past:

Early Observations and Recognition (Late 19th Century)

The early 20th century saw the first recorded observations of what is now known as EDS. Patients with hyperelastic skin and very flexible joints were well-known to doctors. A young infant with hypermobility and hyperelastic skin was described by Danish dermatologist **Edvard Ehlers** in a case report from 1899. This was one of the first instances of EDS that has been documented, even though he didn't name the ailment.

Edvard Ehlers' 1900s Contributions

Cutis hyperelastica (hyperelastic skin), a key research by Edvard Ehlers, was published in the Danish Medical Journal in 1901. This study is often recognized as the foundational work in the development of EDS.

A little girl with hypermobility, hyperelastic skin, and prone to bruising was the subject of Ehlers' investigation. He noted the disease's genetic component.

The Participation of Henri-Alexandre Danlos (1908)

In 1908, Henri-Alexandre Danlos, a French doctor, contributed to our understanding of the illness by presenting a thorough description of what is now known as EDS.

Danlos emphasized the condition's dermatological features, particularly the fragile, easily injured epidermis and joint hypermobility.

Earlier Classification (Twentieth Century)

The condition was known by numerous names in the early 20th century, including "Ehlers-Danlos Syndrome" in honor of both Ehlers and Danlos' groundbreaking research.

The identification of different subtypes, including the classical, hypermobility, and vascular variations, was facilitated by further observations and case reports.

Diagnostic Standards and Genetic Advances in the Late 20th Century

Researchers and physicians developed diagnostic criteria for EDS in the middle to end of the 20th century, enabling more accurate diagnosis and classification.

The hereditary foundation of the condition was revealed by genetic research conducted in the later half of the 20th century that identified unique gene mutations associated with specific EDS subtypes.

Contemporary Understanding (21st Century)

Recent advances in molecular biology and genetic testing have improved our comprehension of EDS. A growing number of genes and genetic pathways linked to the syndrome are being found by researchers. - The exposure and knowledge of EDS have also increased as a result of awareness efforts and patient advocacy initiatives.

The history of Ehlers-Danlos Syndrome is a tribute to the dedication of doctors and scientists who, for more than a century, have slowly and methodically uncovered the mysteries of this complex and diverse group of connective tissue diseases. People with EDS now have more opportunities for early diagnosis, treatment, and support because of improved diagnostic methods and raising awareness.

We have learned a great deal about Ehlers-Danlos Syndrome (EDS) in the 20th century. These developments, which ranged from diagnostic standards to the discovery of genetic markers, were significant turning points in the history of the syndrome.

Identification of Various Subtypes

Researchers and doctors began to realize that EDS included a variety of clinical symptoms around the beginning of the 20th century. As a result, various subtypes including Classical, Hypermobility, and Vascular EDS were named. These subtypes were distinguished by distinctive clinical traits such as skin involvement, joint hypermobility, and vascular fragility.

Creating Diagnostic Criteria

There was an increasing need for standardized diagnostic standards to aid in the identification of EDS during the middle of the 20th century. The Villefranche Classification, which was developed in 1967, provides precise standards for diagnosing and classifying EDS subtypes. This classification system has been widely used and modified throughout time to reflect growing knowledge.

Identification Of Genomic Markers

The latter half of the 20th century saw genomic advances that paved the way for a deeper understanding of the genetic underpinnings of EDS.

A genetic analysis revealed certain mutations connected to different EDS subtypes. For instance, it was shown that the COL5A1 and COL5A2 genes, which encode collagen type V, have the genetic variation linked to Classical EDS.

Molecular insights

Researchers learned more about the molecular mechanisms behind EDS as molecular biology methods advanced. They investigated how the syndrome's usual symptoms are caused by mutations in the genes for connective tissue proteins like collagen. These findings contributed to a better understanding of the abnormal collagen synthesis and structure seen in EDS patients.

New Diagnostic Instruments

The 20th century also saw the introduction of new diagnostic tools, such as genetic testing and electron microscopy, allowing for more precise diagnosis and classification.

   - For example, electron microscopy made it possible to see abnormal collagen fibrils in skin samples from EDS patients.

Awareness and Advocacy

Throughout the 20th century, organizations in medicine and patient advocacy groups dedicated to EDS emerged. These groups were crucial in spreading knowledge, providing assistance, and promoting research.

Early identification and therapy for people with EDS were made possible by greater awareness.

Advances In Treatment And Management

Medical professionals were able to develop more specialized treatment and care procedures for patients because of a better understanding of EDS. This included exercises, methods for managing discomfort, and, in certain cases, surgical operations.

In conclusion, the 20th century was a period of significant growth in our understanding of Ehlers-Danlos Syndrome. These discoveries, which include the categorization of various subtypes, the discovery of genetic markers, and the establishment of diagnostic criteria, have improved the lives of people with EDS by enabling earlier diagnosis and more individualized therapy. Additionally, these developments have laid the foundation for ongoing research and future advancements in the twenty-first century.

Chapter 2

Ehlers-Danlos disorders

A group of rare inherited conditions known as Ehlers-Danlos syndromes (EDS) harm connective tissue.

Skin, tendons, ligaments, blood vessels, internal organs, and bones may all be supported by connective tissues.

Ehlers-Danlos syndrome (EDS) signs and symptoms

Some EDS types may have similar symptoms.

These consist of,

Joint hypermobility or a wider range of joint motion

Stretchy skin

Easily bruised or cracked skin

EDS may have a variety of effects on people. While some people's symptoms may be mild, others may have more serious illnesses.

The many forms of EDS are brought on by genetic flaws that weaken connective tissue.

The faulty gene may have come from one parent or both parents, depending on the kind of EDS.

It's possible for a person to develop a faulty gene without inheriting it.

Some of the severe, rare varieties might be fatal.

Ehlers-Danlos syndromes (EDS) main types

EDS comes in *13 different types*, the majority of which are rare. The kind of EDS that is most common is hypermobile EDS (hEDS).

EDS may also be classified as classical, vascular, or kyphoscoliotic.

Extremely mobile EDS

People who have HEDS may have:

hypermobility of joints

joint pain

clicking joints

Weak, unstable joints that dislocate easily

problems with internal organs, such as mitral valve troubles or organ prolapse

Problems with bladder control (urinary incontinence)

Easily bruised skin

Digestive problems such as indigestion and constipation

Vertigo (losing balance caused by looking down from a greater height)

An accelerated heart rate after rising.

There are no tests available right now to determine whether someone has HEDS.

A person's medical history and a physical examination are used to make the diagnosis.

Traditional EDS

The skin is more often damaged by classical EDS (cEDS), which occurs less frequently than hypermobile EDS.

SIDS sufferers might have:

hypermobility of joints

Stretchy, flimsy skin that is likely to tear easily, especially over the forehead, knees, shins, and elbows, and loose.

unstable joints that dislocate easily

smooth, silky skin that is readily bruised; wounds that take a long time to heal and leave behind a lot of scarring

Prolapsed organs and hernias

Arterial EDS

The unusual form of EDS known as vascular EDS (vEDS) is usually thought to be the most deadly.

Internal organs and blood vessels may get damaged as a result of its effects, which might result in a hemorrhage that could be fatal. People who have vEDS may experience,

Body's bruised skin,notably on the upper chest and legs

The skin is exceedingly thin and clearly shows the presence of little blood vessels.

There is a risk of organ issues such as bowel tearing, womb tearing (in late pregnancy), and partial collapse of the lung

fragile blood vessels that can bulge or tear resulting in serious internal bleeding

hypermobile fingers and toes

unusual facial features (such as a thin nose and lips; large eyes; and small earlobes); varicose veins; and delayed wound healing.

EDS for kyphoscoliosis

It is rare to have kyphoscoliotic EDS (kEDS).

People with KEDS could experience,

Spinal curvature, which starts in early childhood and typically becomes worse in adolescence

As well as joint hypermobility Loose

Flimsy joints that dislocate easily and poor muscle tone
(hypotonia) from birth may delay sitting and walking or make
walking difficult if symptoms become worse

weak eyes that are prone to injury

Bruises easily, scars, and has flexible, velvety skin

Spectrum of hypermobility disorder (HSD)

Some people may have problems brought on by their
hypermobility, but not necessarily one of the specific EDS
illnesses. A diagnosis of hypermobility spectrum disorder (HSD),
which is treated similarly to hEDS, may be made of them.

receiving medical guidance

If you have many bothersome EDS symptoms, see a doctor.

If you just have a few symptoms and they aren't causing any
issues, you usually don't need to worry.

For instance, joint hypermobility affects around 1 in 30 people,
making it fairly common. If you have no additional symptoms,
EDS is unlikely to be the reason.

If your GP suspects that you have EDS and you are experiencing
joint pain, they may refer you to a **rheumatologist**, a specialist in
joints.

The general practitioner may suggest that you visit your local
genetics department for testing if there is a chance that you may
have one of the rare variants of EDS.

A genetic blood test may be performed by the genetics specialist to confirm the diagnosis after asking about your symptoms and medical and family histories.
Your hospital doctor can suggest that you visit a specialist EDS diagnostic service facility if further investigation is necessary.

Chapter 3

Ehlers-Danlos syndrome (EDS) treatment

There is no specific treatment for EDS; however, with support and guidance, many of the symptoms may be managed.

Numerous different healthcare professionals may be able to treat EDS patients.

For instance:

Your joints may be strengthened through **exercise**, which can also help you avoid accidents and manage discomfort.

An occupational therapist can help you manage daily chores and provide guidance on tools that can be helpful.

If you are unable to control long-term discomfort for certain types of EDS, psychotherapy and cognitive behavioral therapy (CBT) may be helpful. Internal organ problems may be found during routine hospital scans.

Genetic counseling may be able to shed further light on the origin of your condition, how it is inherited, and the likelihood that you will pass it on to your offspring.

These services could be suggested by your doctor or consultant.

Ehlers-Danlos syndrome (EDS) affliction

It's important to pay attention to activities that strain your joints or put you at risk of injury.

But it's also important to avoid being too cautious and giving up living a normal life.

Whatever EDS type you have and how it affects you will determine what advice you get.

Some activities, such as contact sports and hard lifting, may be completely discouraged. You may need to wear the proper safety gear and get instructions on how to lessen the pressure on your joints for specific activities. You may be advised to engage in lower-risk activities to help you stay fit and healthy, such as pilates or swimming. If you struggle with weariness, you may learn how to time your activities and preserve energy.

The genetics of Ehlers-Danlos syndromes (EDS)

Although it happens by accident to someone without a family history of the condition, EDS may be inherited.

EDS may be inherited in two main ways

Autosomal dominant inheritance (hypermobile, classical, and vascular EDS): Each of a parent's kids has a one-in-two chance of inheriting the faulty gene that causes EDS.

Autosomal recessive inheritance (kyphoscoliotic EDS): Each of the parents' kids has a 1 in 4 chance of developing the disorder due to the faulty gene being inherited from both parents.

Only the same kind of EDS may be transmitted from one individual to their children.

For instance, a person with hypermobile EDS cannot pass it onto their children.

Within the same family, the illness's severity may vary.

To diagnose Ehlers-Danlos disease genetically.

A range of connective tissue diseases known as Ehlers-Danlos syndrome (EDS) may run in families.

Chapter 4

Ehlers-Danlos syndrome

What is it

Ehlers-Danlos syndrome (EDS) is a term used to describe illnesses that harm your body's connective tissues, which are mostly made of collagen. Bones, muscles, tendons (which form our joints), blood vessels, and the intestines all contain collagen. The skin is also made flexible and durable by collagen.

What possible EDS symptoms may there be?

Chronic joint discomfort (recurring joint pain)

Hypermobile joints (loose, flexible joints)

Orthostatic hypotension (dizziness or lightheadedness while abruptly changing positions)

Simple bruising

Fatigue

supple skin

Strain (striae) markings

The illness is known as Irritable Bowel Syndrome (IBS), which also includes gas, stomach pain, diarrhea, and constipation.

How can EDS spread among families?

A parent's (mother or father) EDS increases the likelihood of each child developing it by 50% (1 out of 2).

A parent's (mother or father) EDS increases the likelihood of each child developing it by 50% (1 out of 2).

The likelihood of each child of an EDS parent also having EDS is 50% (1 out of 2) for the majority of EDS types. Even within the same family, not everyone with EDS experiences the condition in the same way. This is due to the fact that each person's EDS symptoms are unique. Within the same family, the kind of EDS remains the same.

What different types of EDS are there?

EDS may take many different forms; however, these are some of the more common ones:

Type III hypermobility in EDS The most typical EDS is this one. People with this kind have joints that are loose or very flexible and experience joint pain.

Type I and Type II EDS Classic Comparatively fewer people have Type III. These types of EDS exhibit all the symptoms of Type III, as well as brittle, flexible skin, wide scars, and maybe heart issues.

(Type IV) EDS Vascular Type This particular EDS is unusual. Brittle skin, an increased risk of organ rupture (damaging their organs), and blood vessel rupture are all symptoms of type IV diabetes.

How can doctors identify EDS?

Based on your medical history and a physical examination, doctors can determine whether you have EDS. In other words, the geneticist (the genetics physician) will do a physical examination and evaluate your symptoms as well as the flexibility of your joints and skin. The geneticist will also examine your past and the medical background of your family.

What genetic testing options are there for EDS

Depending on the kind of EDS your geneticist suspects you may have, genetic testing for EDS may or may not be available. If testing is provided, health insurance may not pay for it. To find out whether genetic testing is covered by your health insurance, speak with your geneticist or call them.

Genetic testing is not performed if you have EDS Type III, since doctors make this diagnosis based only on a physical examination. At this moment, we are unsure of which gene (a portion of your DNA) accounts for the majority of cases of this kind of EDS.

A blood test is normally available for genetic testing if you have EDS Type I or Type II. However, the genetic test only picks up on around 50% (1 out of 2) of cases. This kind of EDS may also be diagnosed without testing by your geneticist.

If we think you could have EDS type IV, we'll talk to you about getting a genetic test for the COL3A1 gene, which is the culprit in this kind of EDS.

People from all around the world have been showing their support for those who have hypermobility spectrum disorder (HSD) or one of the 13 types of Ehlers-Danlos syndrome (EDS).

Awareness for EDS

Since the first event in 2006, EDS Awareness Month has been held in May under the direction of the Ehlers-Danlos Society.

The Ehlers-Danlos Society may be traced back to 1985, when Nancy Hanna Rogowski founded the Ehlers-Danlos National Foundation (EDNF) in the United States. Nancy founded the EDNF with the intention of uniting people with EDS so that they could provide one another with emotional support. From this simple beginning, the EDNF evolved into a "critical information link." The nonprofit has since helped advance EDS research and public campaigning on a global level.

As "the very first fully global organization committed solely to global research and the support and advocacy for patients, caregivers, and medical professionals," the Ehlers-Danlos Society was established from the former EDNF in May 2016. The group describes EDS Awareness Month as 'a time we all come together, celebrate our growing international community, share experiences, and underline what is necessary to achieve change'.

There have been other fundraising events going on, including the well-known Walk & Roll Challenge. Participants are required to complete a particular distance, whether it be 25 steps, 25 miles, or 250 miles, by walking, running, wheeling, biking, or even using a treadmill! The goal is to collectively cover 25,000 miles, or almost one-third of the Earth's diameter.

#EnoughisEnough

The new #EnoughIsEnough campaign from Ehlers-Danlos Support UK was introduced during EDS Awareness Month. The effort attempts to highlight the fact that people in the UK who have EDS or HSD "have been ignored, causing concern, anguish, and needless agony" with regard to diagnosis and treatment. Ehlers-Danlos Support UK will use community involvement, such as petitions, to pressure the government to increase funding for the NHS in an attempt to address these issues.

Since there is currently no treatment for EDS, therapy focuses on managing the symptoms. Wearing dynamic Lycra® compression clothing, such as those from the Medigarments Ltd. Sensory Dynamic Orthosis (SDO® Original) line, is one approach to achieving this. The clothing may help in a variety of ways, from improving posture and joint stability to reducing pain and enhancing daily functioning.

Chapter 5

Exercise for Ehlers-Danlos syndrome

The importance of exercise is a topic that is often discussed. Rarely a day goes by that we don't hear some expert or another advise us on the news to "get more exercise" and live a healthier lifestyle. I assume your doctor emphasizes exercise every time you see them, and if you ever see a physiotherapist, you can be sure they will promote the benefits of exercise. All of this encouragement to lead a healthy lifestyle and engage in regular exercise is often directed at the whole population, but it is sometimes reserved in particular for groups in society where the benefits are ostensibly greatest.

Unsurprisingly, the evidence supporting the benefits of movement and exercise is utterly overwhelming. In fact, if exercise were available as a medication, it would be the **drug** that was **prescribed** the most all across the globe! What are some of these advantages, then?

Treatment and prevention for the following ailments:

Diabetes

elevated blood pressure

High triglycerides

Heart condition

Obesity

Osteoporosis

Arthritis

both anxiety and depression

These are some of the most prevalent health issues impacting society, and just because you happen to have hypermobility does not excuse you from seeing your doctor or hospital or even from dying each year. There is no guarantee that you won't also acquire hypermobility spectrum disorder (HSD) or Ehlers-Danlos syndrome (hEDS). Exercise may already help protect you from developing the aforementioned conditions, even if it cannot prevent you from having hEDS or HSD.

And working out has extra benefits as well! For illustration:

Having greater confidence going forward

enhancing the body's flexibility in stiff areas so you may go on with your activities

Increasing endurance

enhancing muscle endurance in the body

Release of tension and stress

gaining muscle mass and losing weight Raising fitness levels raising one's self-esteem

We've established the health benefits of exercise, but how can someone who uses hEDS or HSD exercise? One of the most often asked questions by hypermobile patients is this one. They list a variety of problems that might arise after exercise, including **shaky joints**, ongoing pain, postural tachycardia syndrome (POTS), constricted gastrointestinal symptoms, and, of course, tiredness. Exercise (and mobility in general) is a key component of managing hEDS/HSD and may provide you with the opportunity to possibly improve your functional abilities, allowing you to do more in life.

Everyone, yes, everyone, can benefit from exercise and movement. It isn't always easy, and there is a large variety of abilities when it comes to hEDS/HSD and physical conditions ranging from modest to quite severe. The next most frequently asked question is: "What exercise is safe for me to do?" "Are there any exercises that I should avoid?" "How can I avoid deconditioning?" "Should I do stretches?" "How much exercise should I do?" and you simply need to know what type is suitable for you and how to go about it. These are all valid concerns, and this chapter will hopefully address them. However, there are a few crucial issues that must be covered first.

Before beginning any kind of fitness program, you should always make sure that you have received the go-ahead from any doctor you may be under the care of (a cardiologist, gastroenterologist, rheumatologist, general practitioner, etc.). Second, because each person is unique, hEDS/HSD has a different impact on each person. Therefore, there is no substitute for a personal assessment when choosing the best exercise program for you to follow. A completely qualified healthcare expert (a licensed physiotherapist) should ideally do this since they can assess the patient's progress and adjust the exercises as necessary. Since everyone of you will have different needs and physical concerns, it would be difficult to provide an exhaustive list of exercises suitable for everyone in a situation like this. In light of this, everyone should adhere to a few fundamental recommendations when it comes to exercising.

Let's start by taking a closer look at each of the many types of exercise equipment that are available. The main categories exist

Aerobic power flexibility

Proprioception/balance

Aerobic activity

Aerobic power flexibility

Alternatively, it is known as cardiovascular or cardiorespiratory exercise. This exercise stimulates the heart and lungs and transfers oxygen to the muscles. Our normal methods for getting this kind of exercise include walking, using treadmills, exercise bikes, cross-trainers, and swimming, to name a few. The recommended amount in the "normal" population is 150 minutes per week of moderate intensity, broken down into five sessions of 30 minutes each. Even though this may sound like a lot, you may divide each 30 minutes into three 10-minute segments each day, or even six 5-minute segments if you like. What does "moderate intensity" mean? For example, if you are engaging in moderate-intensity exercise, you should be able to talk but not sing during the activity. Some of you may be able to pull this off, in which case go for it! The aforementioned, nonetheless, may be difficult for many of you to achieve as a starting point. Early on, pushing too hard might cause a flare-up. How may it be done more easily or at home? Walking is a great way to get aerobic exercise, as was already said, if you are able. Another strategy is, if you can, to climb and descend steps. What if you have trouble walking? Swimming might be a substitute. You may either swim in the pool or just browse around. No entry to a nearby pool? To "cycle" at home, try buying a tiny pair of free-standing pedals; this may be especially helpful if you have PoTS or are severely under conditioned. You don't need a full-fledged exercise bike. If you have trouble pedaling, you may use the pedals as a handbike by placing them on a table.

Even simple household tasks like cleaning and gardening might count as a kind of cardiovascular exercise. If you are unable to complete 30 minutes each day, don't worry as much. Each and every exercise should be timed, and you should always start with a small, manageable "baseline" amount that you can do without noticeably worsening your symptoms. Start out by doing 5–10 minutes of low-intensity exercise two–three times each week. It's OK. Do what you are capable of. Although it may always be improved, taking action is preferable to doing nothing at all. Despite the fact that it may seem like it uses up all of your energy, cardiac activity may really be a great way to counteract fatigue. As you become fitter, your energy reserves should gradually increase.

Strength training

Exercise of this kind strengthens bones, tendons, ligaments, and muscles. Being stronger increases your joint support and reduces the probability of injury. You are better able to handle physical and functional tasks if you are strong. The following methods of strengthening may be used at home or at a gym:

Use a load of some kind, such as resistance bands, dumbbells, your own body weight, or even gravity. Some suggestions include strengthening your legs by doing sit-to-stand exercises while seated or by placing a resistance band around the back leg of a chair, bringing it forward, putting your foot in it, and then straightening your knee. Carrying a can of beans or a tote bag filled with items while executing bicep curls can help you build stronger arms. Holding a small dumbbell in your hands while raising your arms out to the side can help you build stronger shoulders. If you are prone to subluxations or dislocations, use caution.

As previously stated, start by working out a baseline number of repetitions (reps) per exercise that you feel you can manage without eliciting an exacerbation of your pain (start low) and use a paced approach (even though your pain may be present all the time, we want to avoid anything that really ramps it up and makes it even worse).

Core strength, proprioception, and body awareness may all be improved with Pilates, which are simple mat exercises designed for a therapeutic population. Pilates is also known to assist with motor control. Avoid more advanced traditional Pilates exercises since they may be quite difficult and cause unneeded stress on the body. If you are taking a Pilates class, let the instructor know in advance about your medical situation. The exercises may then be modified by a competent instructor to fit your needs. Verify that the appropriate muscles are working (a physiotherapist's assistance may be very helpful here).

Flexibility

While you are hypermobile, certain parts of you may still feel stiff. Stiffness could be a common problem. Global muscles may regularly overwork themselves and get exhausted, resulting in discomfort and muscle spasms. Keep in mind that pain and inactivity may lead to stiffness, so maintaining flexibility may be beneficial. If we hold static (and unfavorable) postures throughout the day, some parts of our bodies may regularly get stiff. Consider how much time you spend each day lying, standing, or sitting in the same place. It is vital to change postures sometimes because of this. Gentle stretches and "mindful movement," a specific kind of slow, controlled motion, may also help reduce any potential stiffness. Yoga may also be helpful, but be sure to choose a qualified teacher, and please be careful not to overextend yourself into hyperextended postures. The phrase "just because it goes there doesn't mean you should take it there" should be kept in mind! Typically, it could be challenging to figure out where "there" is. It may be difficult to decide when to stop the stretch. Proprioception and balance are the next elements, which are introduced here.

Proprioception and equilibrium

The ability of the body to sense location and movement inside joints is known as proprioception. It enables us to sense the location of our limbs "in space" without having to look. It has to do with coordination. Joints may move out of position as a result of poor joint position sensing. In general, your stability will be greater the stronger your proprioception. How may this be taught at home? There are other possibilities available, but once again, in the absence of an official assessment, your decision will mostly depend on how well you believe you can manage the activity. The most essential thing is to choose a level that is appropriate for you and to provide a safe environment while doing it. Having said that, some options include:

T'ai Chi is a fantastic kind of exercise that involves slow, deliberate movements. beneficial for stability and balance. As well, **Chi Gung** is recommended.

Exercises for balance when standing might include standing with your feet together, doing it while you're **blindfolded**, standing on one leg, or standing on a wobble board. If you're feeling very bold, you might even try doing some tiny squats while standing on a wobble board and throwing and catching a ball.

If you have a Wii Fit, using it to practice stability and balance could be enjoyable. Numerous other games might be added to the Wii Fit board.

The gym ball is a fantastic and versatile piece of home exercise gear. Try adopting good posture when sitting on the ball. Sit down and gradually bring your feet together. If you can, try straightening out one knee and lifting your foot off the ground; if you're feeling very brave, you may do it while keeping your eyes closed.

As previously stated, choosing an exercise that is challenging but not impossible for you is essential when engaging in any form of balance or proprioception exercise. Other safety precautions include exercising on a mat, having chairs placed on either side of you, or standing close to a wall.

It's possible to enjoy exercising; it doesn't have to be a bother. Make sure you have a conducive environment for working out. Avoid the odor of a strenuous exercise by turning on some music or spritzing the space with beautiful scents. Exercise with loved ones or friends to boost motivation. To benefit from exercise and movement, you don't need to belong to a gym. There are a variety of exercises you may do at home, standing or sitting, as was previously mentioned. Just to reiterate, it is usually advised to stay away from contact and/or high-impact activities (for the more courageous among you). Instead, put your attention on proprioceptive training, low- to moderate-impact aerobic activity, and strengthening.

It is still possible and, to be honest, crucial to maintain some level of movement and perform simple exercises yourself at home, even though the best way to develop and adhere to an exercise program is under the supervision of a physiotherapist who will carefully assess your particular needs and be able to monitor and adjust your progress.

Therefore, it is clear that the hypermobile population needs movement and moderate exercise for a variety of reasons. It could help with the pain that comes from deconditioning and stiffness. You could get more energy through exercise to help alleviate fatigue. It might improve your overall stability, reduce your risk of injury, and reduce the number of dislocations you experience. Exercise may also help those of you with POTS lessen their symptoms; just be careful to replenish lost salt afterward with electrolyte drinks or salt tablets taken with water. Exercise may improve mood regulation, produce feel-good hormones like endorphins and encephalins, and reduce anxiety associated with using our bodies via "mindful movement." Exercise improves general fitness and health. Try to think of exercising as a way to help you reach important goals in your life rather than as something you do for its own sake.

The best medicine is undoubtedly exercise.

Chapter 6

What Distinguishes Joint Hypermobility Syndrome From Joint Hypermobility

Hypermobility of the joints is rather common. Your joints may be more mobile than usual if you have hypermobility. Double-jointed is another term that you could hear. This indicates that your joints are quite flexible. The elbows, wrists, fingers, and knees are the joints that are most often affected.

Most people with hypermobility experience no pain or health issues. However, for certain people, hypermobility results in symptoms such as joint discomfort, ligament injuries, weariness, gastrointestinal problems, and others. Young people and children are more prone to the joint hypermobility condition. More often, it affects people of Asian and Afro-Caribbean heritage. It also affects those who are declared female at birth (AFAB). Age usually makes things better.

Is Ehlers-Danlos syndrome the same as joint hypermobility syndrome?

The syndrome of joint hypermobility may be a sign of a more severe underlying genetic condition. Heritable diseases of connective tissue (HDCT) are the names given to these conditions. Joint hypermobility syndrome is associated with the following rare medical conditions:

Your blood, bones, fat, and cartilage are all affected by the illnesses that make up Ehlers-Danlos syndrome. This disorder is brought on by a lack of collagen, a protein that gives your connective tissue flexibility and strength.

Your connective tissue may be damaged by Marfan syndrome. This disorder is brought on by a deficit in the gene that makes elastic and fibrillin fibers, two essential components of your connective tissue.

People with **Down syndrome**, a genetic disorder in which one extra chromosome is present at birth, have abnormal brain and body development.

signs and reasons

How does joint hypermobility syndrome manifest?

Joint and muscular soreness are the most common symptoms of joint hypermobility syndrome. Other signs can include:

frequent injuries to the ligaments and joints, such as sprains and dislocations.

tension in the muscles and joints.

tiredness, or weariness.

Ungainliness/bad balance.

bowel and bladder issues

fainting and dizziness

flexible, thin skin.

What leads to the syndrome of joint hypermobility?

Joint hypermobility syndrome has an unknown origin. But the illness often runs in families. It is believed that the genes involved in collagen production have a purpose. Your joints, ligaments, and tendons are flexible and strong thanks to a protein called *collagen*. Because their ligaments are weak, people with joint hypermobility syndrome have loose joints. Due to a collagen shortage, they have weak ligaments.

Administration and Therapy

How is the syndrome of joint hypermobility treated?

The condition of joint hypermobility is now untreatable. Protecting your joints and managing your pain are part of the treatment. By enhancing your muscular strength through exercise, you can protect your joints. Additional ideas include:

Keep good posture.

Avoid extreme ranges of motion by standing with your knees slightly bent.

Put on supportive, arch-supporting footwear.

To help fix flat feet, use orthotics.

To lessen pain, increase muscle strength, and optimize your posture and balance, see a physical therapist.

Your doctor could recommend an over-the-counter pain reliever, such as acetaminophen (Tylenol®), ibuprofen (Advil®, Motrin®), or naproxen (Aleve®), for minimal discomfort. Your healthcare provider could recommend stronger painkillers or provide additional treatments to help you manage your pain if it is more severe.

How can I prevent the syndrome of joint hypermobility?

A genetic disorder called joint hypermobility syndrome often runs in families. Because of this, it cannot be halted.

If I have joint hypermobility syndrome, what can I expect?

Children and teens are the age groups most often affected by joint hypermobility syndrome. The severity of symptoms seems to decrease with age. Other people just have slight symptoms. Others may experience intense discomfort. It's important to discuss ways to protect your joints and manage your discomfort with your healthcare provider.

What is the diet for joint hypermobility syndrome

According to research, gastrointestinal problems, including irritable bowel syndrome (IBS), and hypermobility may be related. Joint hypermobility syndrome is a common cause of IBS symptoms. Therefore, to check for an intolerance to certain food components, your healthcare provider may suggest an exclusion diet. Your symptoms could go away if whatever is causing the intolerance is taken care of.

The following are the top three exclusion diets:

Diet without gluten

To determine whether you are allergic to gluten, gluten is removed from your diet.

Diet without lactose

To determine whether you are sensitive to dairy products, lactose is removed from your diet.

Low-FODMAP diet

You cut out a group of five sugars that are found in certain foods. These sugars include galactans, fructans, lactose, fructose, and polyols. Fermentable oligosaccharides, disaccharides, monosaccharides, and polyols are referred to as FODMAP.

How can I look after myself?

Maintaining a healthy lifestyle is essential if you have joint hypermobility syndrome in order to protect your joints. Regular exercise may help you strengthen your muscles and joints.

-

    Taking regular breaks while working out

-

consuming a balanced diet.

- putting on supportive footwear.

- Warm baths may relieve joint pain and stiffness.

- Not deliberately overextending your joints.

A connective tissue ailment called joint hypermobility syndrome Many people have very flexible joints or have multiple joints. However, joint hypermobility syndrome may be the cause when you also have painful joints and other symptoms. In addition to a physical examination, a test or questionnaire on your flexibility is used to diagnose joint hypermobility syndrome. Although there is no cure, maintaining healthy joints and taking medication may help to reduce symptoms. If you encounter severe symptoms, see your healthcare provider.

They may aid in your illness management.